HEARTS OF HEALTH

A Heart Nurse's Guide to Health
in the 21st Century
By
Alicia Lown, R.N.

alicialown.com

In Gratitude

I AM Grateful to Cynthia Jordan for all the inspiration, encouragement and help she has offered me throughout the years. This book would not have happened without her.

I AM Grateful to my editors Kathryn Louie and Diane Mobley.

I AM Grateful to my friend Bill Worrell for the beautiful Heart cover art for the book and for ALL the amazing art he has created over the years.

I AM Grateful to my friend Patch Adams, M.D., for his inspiration and his endless efforts to spread Peace, Happiness, Joy, and Health throughout the world.

I AM Grateful to my "Amorgo" Darren Morrison for supporting me throughout this healing journey.

I AM Grateful to my Yogic Family.

I AM Grateful to my animal family Chula, Sister Bobbie, Dolly Pawton, Panchita, Shakey, Augustus McCrea aka "Gus", Edna, and Rosie. They have brought me much joy over the years.

I AM Grateful to my family, special thanks to my brother Joseph Lown for his constant support and encouragement.

I AM Grateful to my Creator and all my many blessings.

DEDICATION

*In Memory of my parents
George and Alicia Lown*

CONTENTS

1

MY STORY

I grew up pretty much smack dab in the Heart of Texas. Yep, I'm a true Texan...I rode cutting horses, I say *y'all*, I LOVE Willie Nelson and *Lonesome Dove* is one of my all-time favorite movies. My father was half Swedish and my mother was half Mexican. She was actually born and raised in Mexico City, which was the largest city in the world at the time. They met and fell in love in Vienna, Austria, while traveling through Europe with mutual friends. My parents were a bit of an odd couple. Physically my dad was a rather large man who had a very large, outgoing personality. In contrast, my mother was petite, prim, and proper. Their marriage seemed to work out for a while, about 22 years or so, but they divorced after my dad was diagnosed with congestive heart failure. I was in nursing school at the time.

My dad was a big man and when I say big, I mean BIG. He was over six feet tall and at one point tipped the scales at 416 pounds. He also had a huge heart, was gregarious and fun loving, and loved to tell jokes. He was born fat and actually came out of the womb a chubby baby. Throughout his life, his weight ranged from slightly overweight to morbidly obese. For a while, there was only one scale in town on which he could weigh himself, and that was at the local animal feed store! If you have ever heard the country song "I was country when country wasn't cool," well "He was fat, when fat wasn't cool." This was back in the 70's and 80's, before two-thirds of our country was overweight.

I'm not going to lie…it was not easy growing up with a fat dad. At times I was flat out embarrassed about it. But mainly, due to his weight and poor health, he never really felt like spending quality time with us. I would have enjoyed having more time playing sports and being outdoors with him. I was extremely active and, while growing up, loved to play all sports. I was the only girl on the flag football and basketball team in third grade and would have played tackle football if the powers that be would let me.

My dad was on a diet his ENTIRE life! When I was in junior high, he once went on a diet where he did not eat any food for an entire year! He drank only "shakes" and took vitamins. He lost over 100 lbs. and looked so different that his own mother did not even recognize him. But unfortunately the weight loss was only temporary, as he proceeded to gain it all back, PLUS about another 100 lbs.

My 95-year-old Swedish cousin tells me how my dad's parents thought it was "cute" to stuff him with food. Needless to say, my dad's dad died in his 40's of a massive heart attack when my dad was only 12 years old. His brother, my dad's uncle, also died in his early 50's of a massive heart attack. From what I understand, they burned the candle at both ends. The fact that my dad lived to the ripe age of 62 was pretty amazing, considering his doctors could not believe that he went on as long as he did with a heart as weak as it was. I'll tell you what, *where there's a will there's a way*! This man loved people and loved life. He actually died of cardiomegaly, which is an enlarged heart, and he definitely had a large heart in more ways than one.

My mom, on the other hand, was a beautiful petite senorita. She reached all of about 5'1" and 110 lbs. and spoke perfect Spanish and English. My mom was never overweight or hardly sick a day in her life, well until she died of breast cancer when she was only 53 years old. No one would have ever guessed that my dad would outlive my mom. All who knew her were truly shocked to hear of her passing. My mother was a lovely lady; she was beautiful with light skin and hazel eyes. To this day, over 20 years after her passing, people still come up to me and tell me how beautiful and kind she was.

My mother was an entrepreneur and a strong businesswoman. She became a paralegal assistant after coming to the States and then went on to get her real estate license to become a real estate broker. She was active in the community and was involved in Toastmasters and the Rotary Club.

She was NOT, however, a homemaker. She rarely ever cooked. My brother and I literally grew up on the "SAD DIET" (the Standard American Diet that consists of mainly processed, artificial, and chemically modified junk food). Her idea of cooking might be popping a tortilla with cheese in the toaster oven. We ate out almost every meal. A good meal for us might be going to our local deli, Mr. T's, and getting a BBQ sandwich or going over to our next door neighbor's restaurant, Southern Seas, and having fried fish with greasy bread puffs oozing with honey. Our family ate at about every joint in town! Everybody knew us. My dad usually knew what he wanted and would sometimes order before he ever sat down. By the time I was just a few bites into my meal, he would be finished with his and "eyeballing" my plate. The joke between my brother and me was, when anyone asked us what George was up to, we would joke, "Breakfast, Lunch, and Dinner!" Bless his heart, he was truly larger than life!

My first job as a teenager was at an old-fashioned drugstore on Main Street in San Angelo,

Texas, called Hudman Drug Store. We were known for selling nickel-a-dip ice cream cones. My job title was "Soda Jerk," which translates today as waiting tables, preparing food, and serving ice cream cones, shakes, malts, and banana splits. It was truly a dream job for a kid. The perks included all the ice cream I could eat…and cherry Dr. Peppers, made with real cherry syrup, and grilled ham and cheese sandwiches. I was truly blessed! For five years I ate ice cream and drank all the cokes I wanted at least six days a week. And my parents did not have to worry about feeding me, although they did have to worry about taking me to the dentist often. That is how I ended up with a mouth full of mercury amalgam fillings, which I later had to have removed due to mercury poisoning!

It is no wonder I did not turn into 2-Ton Tess in those five years. I was very fortunate to work with two amazing pharmacists and mentors, whom I adored. They were two of the finest gentlemen around. I supposed this was my first experience working in the "health care industry." I watched them push LOTS of drugs in those five years.

After high school, I went on to nursing school and by 22 years old, I was pushing lots of drugs myself in the cardiac unit at the local hospital. Although I loved the connection with all the patients and other health care providers, I soon found that taking care of critically ill heart patients was extremely stressful and downright scary at times. Rushing around passing out loads of medications of which I barely understood their actions and interactions, just was not my cup of tea.

After about a year, I was transferred to the rehab unit, which turned out to be a great move. One, I did not have to pass out loads of drugs; the LVN's did that. Two, we worked very closely together as a team with the patients, doctors, physical therapists, occupational therapists, speech therapists, social workers, recreational therapists, and the families to see that each patient had great individualized care. This team effort really helped to facilitate a good healing experience for each patient. I learned a lot working in the rehab unit and found it very rewarding.

I next moved on to home health care. I enjoyed getting out in the community and seeing patients in their homes. This kind of nursing gave me a chance to connect with patients on a true level. It was also fun for a while, but the Medicare guidelines required PILES of paperwork for the RN's. Sitting at a desk and doing tons of paperwork was not my strong point either. I wanted a more intimate connection with patients.

Our hospital had a great health club, where I enjoyed working out frequently. I began to notice a program that was offered called Cardiac Rehabilitation. I soon realized this was my *dream* nursing job, and before long, a position became available and I got the job. Working out of a gym and helping people recover after a cardiac event, whether the event be open-heart surgery, heart attack, heart blockage or congestive heart failure, was exactly what I wanted to be doing. We would first see people as inpatients in the hospital and start them on a walking and education program. Then, once they were home and stable enough, they would begin Phase 2 of the program that involved coming to the gym three times per week for a monitored exercise and education program. We would educate them on areas of nutrition, stress management, home exercise, and healthy lifestyle habits.

As a nurse working in such a fun and positive atmosphere…I absolutely loved it. Soon I was promoted to Cardiac Rehab Coordinator. Seeing people heal from heart disease and adopt new, positive, and healthy lifestyles was so fulfilling. This kept me on my game and also made me take good care of myself. This was a fun job and very rewarding as we really became close to these folks. We had lots of laughs, too!

One night, when I was home watching E-Entertainment TV, a program came on about the top 10 cities in the United States to live. It featured a city named Eugene, Oregon. They showed footage of its farmers market, where many of the locals flock each week to buy their fresh grown fruits and vegetables. I was absolutely blown away because I had never seen so many beautiful, colorful berries and vegetables in my life. Rows and rows of them! I did not even know events like this took place.

There was live music, local artisans, handmade clothing, and *delicious* food…AND it was all grown and made locally.

I immediately sought out a way to get to Eugene, Oregon. I found out that nurses could sign on with traveling nurse agencies. These agencies would set nurses up with a home and job virtually anywhere in the US. I was on it and soon was driving west to Eugene, Oregon, with a few personal belongings, my clothes, and my cat.

Eugene is the home of the University of Oregon and the Oregon Ducks. It is the second largest city in Oregon. It is a beautiful city with two rivers running through it and lots and lots of trees. I had never seen so much natural beauty and greenery in all my life.

I worked at Sacred Heart Medical Center, mainly in the Cardiac/Telemetry Unit. I made lots of friends at the hospital; actually I think most of them just got a kick out of my Southern accent. I soon introduced myself to the staff at the Cardiac Rehab Unit, and after completing my 6-month contract, was hired as a Cardiac Rehab Nurse. I was once again immersed in what I like to call True Health Care. Our patients seemed to always improve, lose weight, feel better, and appeared less stressed and much happier.

This program in Oregon was really awesome. A majority of the staff were exercise physiologists, so they really knew their stuff and walked their walk. They even offered Yoga and Tai Chi for their patients, which wasn't mainstream back in 2000. This was my first experience around Yoga and 11 years later I became a certified Kundalini yoga instructor, which by the way was probably one of the best moves I ever made. To this day I still practice and teach yoga. I have gained many benefits from yoga, as well as a very strong support system of wonderful people.

As fate would have it, I ended up falling in love and getting engaged to a fellow who was a fiddle player. He was from Louisiana originally. We would often reminisce of our love for the South, and before long we were loaded up and headed to Texas. Our destination was Austin, Texas, in hopes that he would land a great music career there. I once again got a wonderful job as a cardiac rehab nurse at North Austin Medical Center. Life was good for a while, but breaking into the Austin music scene was not as easy as expected. It was also at this time that I began to get these strange bouts of what seemed to be "food poisoning" with severe vomiting.

After several years of trying to make a go of the Austin music scene, we decided to move back to Oregon. I was very fortunate to get my old job back in the Cardiac Rehab Department at Sacred Heart Hospital. But over the next year or two, the horrible bouts of vomiting became more frequent, to the point I was vomiting pure bile. These bouts would sneak up on me, and I never knew when it was going to happen. I began to get scared and at one point I thought I might have stomach cancer or something just as terrible. Fortunately, a gastroenterologist with whom I worked talked me out of that crazy notion.

I was given a recommendation to see a husband/wife team of nutritional Ph.D.'s. After a long assessment, they determined that I had a whole

16

slew of things going on with me, including adrenal fatigue, low stomach acid production, liver and gall bladder issues, and to top it off, mercury and arsenic poisoning. I was completely blown away. This was all so foreign to me, since I had always been strong and healthy. I was given tons of supplements to take and a diet to follow, which included eating foods like beets and leafy greens to help cleanse and nourish my gall bladder and liver. Previously my diet had consisted of large amounts of processed wheat products, grains, dairy, eggs, and pasta…and occasionally some fresh fruits and veggies from the farmers market.

Around that time, I also began getting unusual skin rashes. Things really were not improving and the vomiting was getting worse. Once it started, I would be vomiting for hours. It was AWFUL! I felt as if my life was coming down around me. My engagement fell apart, I lost a good friend to a falling out, and my gut and health were a wreck.

I truly thought I was a healthy person before all this. The only ailment I ever had was when I was about 27 years old I developed what doctors called rosacea. Horrible, untimely flushing in my face and ears that was set off by numerous triggers such as emotions, hot or spicy foods, alcohol, heat, direct sunlight... you name it. It was a terrible inconvenience. Doctors still have not learned what really causes rosacea.

I went from having a beautiful complexion and never needing to wear makeup, to constantly worrying about powdering my nose and covering up this extreme redness. My face would overheat at the drop of a hat and I would look like a ripe tomato. Later in my 30's the flushing went into my feet, another real inconvenience.

With all of my mysterious health issues, I finally decided it was time to head back home to my roots in Texas and take some time off to heal. My brother had bought a beautiful property on 10 acres in Christoval, Texas, and this was where I spent the next eight years healing, searching, studying, and learning. I was immersed in nature and gardening, which soon proved to be a great healer for me.

I found a local doctor of integrative medicine who helped me to detox and remove the mercury and heavy metal poisoning from my body. He had me arrange to have all the mercury fillings removed from my teeth and started me on IV chelation to remove the rest of the toxins that were poisoning me.

Having mercury fillings removed can be a potentially dangerous procedure, especially all at once. If you decide to go this route, please be aware of the danger and have a good doctor and dentist who know what they are doing. My doctor prescribed supplements to take and a diet to follow. Eventually I started getting better. I have not had a bout with vomiting in over seven years. Thank you!!! Thank you!!!

Since this health crisis, I have been studying and implementing everything I can get my hands on related to health, wellness, happiness, and nutrition. I have tried about every fad diet that has come along. If you name it, I probably have tried it. I have seen multiple doctors and health care practitioners of all sorts and have spent thousands and thousands of dollars on my search for health and wellness.

The following are just a FEW of the treatments I have tried on my quest back to health: Eastern medicine, western medicine, northern medicine (dipping my face in ice water), southern living (moved to Hawaii to live and work at an eco-resort), Chinese medicine, Ayurvedic medicine, Panchakarma, raw food retreats, bulletproof diet (drinking buttered coffee), Reiki, energy medicine, oneness blessing, naturopathy, iridology, candida treatments, Chakra therapy, nutritionist, functional medicine, alternative medicine, integrative medicine, chiropractic, crystal therapy, essential oils, yoga, weight training, salt therapy, meditation, angel therapy, prayer, counseling, Matrix energetics, past life regression, a Course in Miracles, liver/gall bladder flushes, biofeedback, silver therapy, music therapy, meditation, breathing exercises, Chinese herbs, American herbs, healing touch, reflexology, acupuncture, affirmations, guided imagery, forgiveness techniques, Bach flower remedies, nature walks, walking meditations, silent retreats, Tibetan sound healing, positive thinking, tapping techniques, Silva mind training, and genetic testing and treatment…and the list goes on! I know, I know, it's over the top!

In hindsight, I realize there were several areas in my life that were out of balance during my younger years.

1. My relationship with my parents, especially with my mother, was a rocky one. The state of our relationships with our parents usually carries out into all our other relationships.

2. After I left Texas to explore greener grasses, I was no longer following a regular exercise program.

3. I knew very little about eating healthy food and proper nutrition.

4. My faith and spiritual practice was lacking as well.

Years of trial and error were taken to discover the keys to health and happiness. I was usually searching outside myself for all the answers. The answers began to come when I turned and looked within.

Through my experiences and personal quest for health and happiness, I am excited to share with you these tips to staying healthy in the 21st Century! Thanks for listening to my story and being here. Here is a toast to our health and happiness.

2

RAINBOWS AND FOOD

Let us start with food, since I feel passionately that this kind of information would have saved my parents lives. What we put in our mouths is vital to our health. You are what you eat. It is true! The foods we eat make up and nourish our bodies, cells, organs, and blood. When we eat nourishing foods such as fruits, vegetables, and whole foods, we look and feel better. But when we eat junky, artificial, and chemically modified Frankenfoods (ingredients that have been processed in a lab), well you guessed it…we probably are not going to look and feel so great.

It is really this simple. Eating colorful fruits and vegetables, like in the colors of the rainbow, provide us with the essential nutrients we need to thrive, and even to heal disease.

Make Roy G. Biv your new best friend. This is a handy little acronym to remember the colors of the rainbow.

The R in Roy is for red:
Apples
Cherries
Pomegranates
Radishes
Raspberries
Red bell pepper
Red butter lettuce
Strawberries
Watermelon

O is for Orange:
Apricots
Butternut squash
Cantaloupe
Carrots
Mangos
Oranges
Papayas

24

Peaches
Persimmons
Pumpkin
Sweet Potatoes
Yams

Y is for yellow:
Bananas
Lemons
Pears
Pineapple
Squash
Yellow Bell Peppers

G is for green:
Artichokes
Asparagus
Avocados
Bok choy
Broccoli
Brussel sprouts
Butter lettuce
Cabbage

Celery
Cilantro
Cucumbers
Herbs
Kale
Leafy greens
Limes
Romaine lettuce
Spinach
Sprouts
Swiss chard

B is for Blue and I is for Indigo:
Blueberries - Wild blueberries are 100 times stronger than conventional blueberries!

And finally V is for violet:
    Eggplant (they come in violet too)
    Grapes
    Lavender
    Plums
    Purple cabbage
    Purple potatoes

Each of these colorful fruits and vegetables provide different nutrients and antioxidants. Antioxidants fight off free radicals/oxidation, helping us thrive and heal. Adding as many different fruits and vegetables as possible to your diet will be beneficial to your health. Antioxidants from fruits and vegetables are the best Fountain of Youth out there!

Here are some helpful tips:

1. Take time to chew your food well.
2. Give thanks for all this wonderful food as it nourishes your body.
3. The best beverage is good old H_2O. Adding lemon or lime to water promotes hydration and gently cleanses the body and major organs such as the liver.

Remember, too, that our bodies require sodium for proper cell function and the right kind of salt matters. Himalayan pink salt is one of my favorite salts, it is loaded with 84 active minerals. Celtic sea salt is another healthy choice. A *very* small amount of salt is all we need. When possible, choosing foods with natural sodium is best. Some foods that contain natural sodium are spinach, avocado, sweet potatoes, and celery. Celery is actually a miracle food; it is packed with mineral salts that fuel the body and brain. Drinking celery juice alone on an empty stomach will help rebuild hydrochloric acid in the stomach and promote healthy digestion.

Nuts and seeds are convenient to carry and make for a healthy snack. Because of their high fat content, a little bit goes a long way. In fact a small handful is sufficient. My favorites are macadamia nuts, pecans, walnuts, sunflower seeds, cashews, hemp seeds, and pistachios.

Raw fruits and vegetables such as apples, oranges, dates, celery, carrots, and bananas also make great snacks. Grocery stores even carry rainbow-colored carrot sticks now! I find if I have healthy snacks around, I am less likely to get "hangry" and reach for junk food.

The grazing method of eating, which is eating small amounts of fruits and vegetables every couple of hours, is one of the best ways to support our bodies and adrenal glands. When we skip meals frequently and go for long periods without eating, this forces the adrenal glands to kick in and release adrenaline, which is corrosive to the body and drains the adrenal glands.

3

FOODS TO AVOID

The top 5 problematic foods:
Corn
Dairy
Eggs
Soy
Wheat

We are all individuals, so keep in mind that what may be healthy for one person may be toxic and harmful for the next. Sadly, now that corn and soy are mostly genetically modified, they have been proven to be unhealthy. Dairy and eggs are packed with saturated fats, cholesterol and feed pathogens such as harmful viruses and bacteria. If you are trying to heal from any condition, it is best to avoid these foods. Nature intended dairy to be for baby cows and other animals, not for human consumption. Humans are the only species that drink the milk of other mammals! When I eliminated these foods from my diet, my excess fluff came right off, my overall health improved significantly, and I felt great!

A few other foods to be aware of that could be toxic to your health are hydrogenated and partially hydrogenated oils such as vegetable oil, canola oil, corn oil, and margarine. The process used to produce these oils makes them toxic and inflammatory to the body. Using oils *sparingly* or avoiding them altogether is highly recommended. Following a diet low in fats and high in fruits and vegetables will lower blood pressure, cleanse the liver and other organs, lower cholesterol, and can even reverse heart disease and Type 2 diabetes.

Be cautious when eating anything that comes out of a box. Unfortunately cereals, which we once believed to be healthy foods, fall into this category. There was a time in my life when cereal made up two out of my three meals on some days. These foods are "processed," meaning they are typically stripped of their original form and then replaced with additives, preservatives, and sugars to make them taste like food again. They have a long shelf life due to the abundance of additives and preservatives in them. I like to call these foods "Frankenfoods", which I referred to earlier. A healthier alternative to boxed cereals would be natural oatmeal.

Processed foods can be found in the center aisles of the grocery store and are in boxes or packages. Artificial and "natural" ingredients usually make up these foods. I recommend avoiding products with any artificial sweeteners and coloring, refined sugars, and flavors like MSG (MSG is often hidden under the "natural flavors" label).

Learn to read labels. The more ingredients listed in a product (especially the ones you cannot pronounce), the more processed and artificial the food. Instead, choose foods with easily recognized ingredients. If you don't know what's in it, don't eat it!

Due to our busy lives, many have turned to fast food. Fast foods typically fill us with the lowest quality, most unhealthy food for the buck. When you can, go for the freshest options such as salads, fresh vegetables, and small amounts of quality lean meats.

Pastas and breads are considered processed foods. Whole-wheat foods, which were once considered to be some of the healthiest food choices out there, are now controversial. The wheat we grow now in the United States is not the same wheat your mother and grandmother ate. Due to hybridization and mass production, wheat now has much higher amounts of gluten, which is a protein. Gluten can be difficult to digest for many, hence the rise of celiac disease and gluten intolerance. Also wheat feeds pathogens in the body and turns straight to sugar in the bloodstream. In my experience, avoiding wheat products is best if you have any health conditions or are trying to lose weight.

My dad was a diet soda fanatic. If he was not drinking diet sodas, he was drinking iced tea loaded up with artificial sweeteners. I am not sure I ever saw him drink water. These drinks sure did not seem to help him lose weight either. Recent studies now have shown that diet sodas and artificial sweeteners are in no way, shape, or form, good for our health. They do not promote weight loss. In fact, diet sodas can actually cause weight retention and weight gain!

Animal foods such as meats, chicken, fish, eggs, and dairy products sadly have few health benefits for humans. One of the most comprehensive studies on this was *The China Study*, conducted by T. Colin Campbell, Ph.D., the Jacob Gould Schurman Professor Emeritus of Nutritional Biochemistry at Cornell University, and his son Thomas M. Campbell, M.D.

The China Study examined the relationship between the consumption of animal products (including dairy) and chronic illnesses such as coronary heart disease, diabetes, breast cancer, prostate cancer, and bowel cancer. The doctors concluded that people who eat a whole-food, plant-based vegan diet – avoiding all animal products, including beef, pork, poultry, fish, eggs, cheese, and milk – and reducing their intake of processed foods and refined carbohydrates will escape, reduce, or reverse the development of numerous diseases. They write, "eating foods that contain any cholesterol above 0 mg is unhealthy".

I am not saying to give up all your animal foods but to do your own research and to learn for yourself. For me, since I have adopted a mostly plant-based vegan diet over the last two years, I have experienced many health benefits, including weight loss, stabilized blood sugars, optimal cholesterol levels, and fewer allergies and skin rashes. The book and documentary *Forks over Knives* has been a great resource for many who want to learn more about plant-based foods. They have a great app that can be used to help plan, shop, and prepare healthy meals.

You can also check out the *meatlessmonday.com* movement. The movement has spread to 44 countries worldwide! Skipping meat one day a week is not only good for your health but also the health of the planet.

4

SHOPPING TIPS

When I first moved to Oregon, one of my favorite pastimes was finding all the small local mom-and-pop grocery stores. I was amazed by all the beautiful farm fresh fruits, vegetables, and colorful displays. Eating healthy seemed to be a way of life there. Local farmers would invite people to come out to their "U Pick" farms and harvest delicious blueberries, raspberries, and strawberries. There is nothing quite like picking and eating fruit straight from the vine.

I suggest sticking to the outer perimeter of the grocery store when shopping. This is the best way to end up with a basket full of healthy fruits and vegetables. I prefer to buy organic produce when available.

Strive for buying one-ingredient foods, rather than packaged or prepared foods with multiple ingredients. Getting a variety of colorful fruits and vegetables is always a plus. Try out new foods and recipes each week – be experimental. Getting to know your produce staff is helpful, too. These folks are usually very knowledgeable and will even special order items for you.

I had never even heard of bok choy until I was in Nutrition and Health Coaching School. We learned that bok choy is in the cruciferous family and is loaded with many great nutrients. There are two main varieties of bok choy: baby bok choy and regular bok choy. This vegetable is like two veggies in one, since the tops are leafy green and the bottoms are white, crispy and juicy! They go great in stir-fries or just plain sautéed or steamed up by themselves.

If possible when buying meats, buy local, grass fed, organic, or pasture raised meats. Although I recommend very little or no animal products for optimum health, I feel better choosing meats that were raised sustainably without added hormones and antibiotics. It also does my heart good to know that these animals were possibly treated better and were able to graze on *real foods*. Americans are in no way, shape, or form deficient in protein; we are, however, lacking in fiber from fruits and vegetables!

Once again, try to stay away from the processed foods in the center section of the grocery store. This is where those crazy Frankenfoods hide out. Our foods should not be concocted in laboratories. Let's keep it real y'all!

Hey, if you do happen to eat a big ice cream cone or a greasy pizza on occasion, go ahead and enjoy every bite of it. Feeling guilty about our food choices does *not* do our body and mind any good.

5

THE DIRTY DOZEN
AND THE CLEAN 15

The Environmental Working Group has created two lists of produce they refer to as the *Clean 15* and the *Dirty Dozen. The Clean 15* are foods with the least contamination of pesticides. The *Dirty Dozen* has the highest amounts of pesticide residue.

When possible, buy organic. If you do buy fruits and veggies on the *Dirty Dozen* list, wash and soak these foods thoroughly. Add 1 cup of apple cider vinegar to 2-3 liters of water and soak 5 minutes.

Here are the *Clean 15* and *Dirty Dozen* lists provided by the Environmental Working Group. You can see the full list on the Environmental Working Group website www.ewg.org

MOST CONTAMINATED FOODS	LEAST CONTAMINATED FOODS
Apples	Asparagus
Celery	Avocados
Cherries	Cabbage
Grapes	Cantaloupe
Nectarines	Cauliflower
Peaches	Eggplant
Pears	Grapefruit
Potatoes	Honeydew Melon
Spinach	Kiwi
Strawberries	Mangoes
Sweet bell peppers	Onions
Tomatoes	Papayas
	Pineapples
	Sweet corn
	Sweet peas (frozen)

6

FARMERS MARKET

Getting to know your local farmers can be a great experience. I love spending Saturday mornings at the local farmers market. Spending time at the market is also a great family outing; teaching and involving children early on about healthy food is important. Like the farmers market I was drawn to in Oregon, many farmers markets have delicious food, arts and crafts, and entertainment.

Our local farmers market has native plants for purchase as well. One of my favorite farmers is a local doctor who raises all of his produce organically. He even sells his own line of herbs and spices. Herbs and spices have been used for eons for medicinal and cooking purposes. For instance, parsley is a great cleansing herb, as it pulls out toxins from our bodies and cleanses the kidneys. Cilantro will actually draw out heavy metals like mercury from the body. Oregano and thyme are powerful natural antibiotics, as is garlic.

Another local farmer jokes that her produce is all organic except for the city water! She is the one that got me hooked on figs. This past summer I discovered how much I loved homegrown apricots and figs, both of which are full of nutrients. Yummy! I have also made friends in the past with hunters. They typically love to share their fresh game with others. Venison stew with lots of veggies makes for a wonderful low fat meal.

7

GROW YOUR OWN GARDEN

If you are concerned about the expense of eating organic and buying fresh fruits and veggies, consider growing your own garden. It does not take much room and seeds are cheap. If you have no experience in gardening, there are some excellent books to help get you started. One is called *Square Foot Gardening* by Mel Bartholomew, which teaches how to grow a garden with limited space. Go to your local nursery and talk with them about organic gardening, they can help get you started as well.

I was so inspired by all the delicious homegrown fruits and vegetables at the local farmers market, I planted seven different fruit trees in my small yard this fall, including two varieties of plums, a nectarine, an apricot, a fig, an apple, a peach, and a pear.

I was concerned about watering them with city water for several reasons: 1) the expense and 2) the chlorine and fluoride added to city water. To handle this concern, I put in rain gutters and a 250-gallon tank. So far I have had plenty of rainwater to get the trees going…and I live on the edge of the Chihuahuan Desert! A little rain goes a long way when it is harvested correctly. The next things on my list to plant are pomegranates, goji berries, and blueberry bushes.

One great perk of gardening is that getting your hands and feet in the dirt is actually beneficial to the body, mind, and immune system. AND the other added benefit is that working outdoors, you are getting your share of Vitamin D, one of the vitamins we are most likely to be deficient in. By growing your own food you can enjoy all the benefits of improved health and immunity plus all the delicious fruits and veggies you can eat!

8

RECIPES

GREEN SMOOTHIE

1 c. water

½ small avocado (optional, makes for nice texture)

1 banana

1 c. frozen fruit – peaches, pineapple, mangoes, or apricots

2 handfuls leafy greens – spinach, kale, romaine, or your favorite lettuce or greens mix. Add in a couple sprigs of your favorite herbs, if desired – mint, cilantro, or basil.

Optional: Add 1-2 tbsp. chia, hemp, or flax seeds. (I like to add the seeds at the very end so I can still get the chewing effect. This helps digestion.)

Blend ingredients in a blender and ENJOY!

Smoothies are an excellent way to start the day and they make a healthy snack.

BERRY BLUE SMOOTHIE

1 c. water

½ small avocado (optional)

1 c. frozen wild blueberries (wild blueberries have the highest antioxidants of all foods!)

1 banana, fresh or frozen

2 handfuls of leafy greens – spinach, kale, romaine, or your favorite lettuce or greens mix. Add in several sprigs of your favorite herbs, if desired – mint, cilantro, or lemon balm

Optional – 1- 2 tbsp. Hemp seeds

Blend ingredients in a blender and ENJOY!

(For a low-fat version, reduce or omit the avocado and hemp seeds)

EASY PEASY STIR FRY

½ lb. lean organic ground beef, turkey, or venison
(Vegetarians use: 2 c. mushrooms. I like shitakes)
1 tsp. coconut oil and 1 tsp. sesame oil
½ onion, chopped
2-3 garlic cloves, chopped
4 c. veggies, including red or green cabbage, bell peppers (red, orange, or yellow), peas, bok choy, mung bean sprouts, carrots, and broccoli.
Seasonings: sea salt, red pepper, ginger (fresh or powdered), cilantro, and coconut aminos. I like *Coconut Secret*, a gluten free soy sauce alternative.

Cook meat and set aside. Add oil (or water for lower fat version) and onions/mushrooms and sauté for a few minutes on medium heat. Then add vegetables and cook for several minutes until desired texture (I prefer mine less cooked to preserve nutrients). Put in the meat that had been set aside and the desired seasonings. Cook another minute or so. Serve with freshly chopped cilantro.

BLACK BEAN SPINACH SALAD

1 box/package organic spinach
1 can (15 oz.) black beans, drained and rinsed (or freshly cooked)
1 handful cilantro, chopped
¾ c. cherry tomatoes, sliced
1 sliced avocado
½ chopped red, orange, or yellow bell pepper
Purple onion, sliced (optional)

Mix all ingredients in a bowl and season with a dash of cumin powder, sea salt, pepper, a dash of olive oil (optional) and your favorite vinegar (optional). Top with a squeeze of fresh lime. Mmmm! This salad is loaded with plant based proteins!

BLACK BEAN KALE & CACTUS SOUP

1 16 oz. package black beans
1 large onion, chopped
6-8 cloves garlic, diced
1 can diced tomatoes
3 large carrots, chopped
2 stalks celery, chopped
¼ tsp. cumin powder
2 tbsp. chili powder, 1 diced jalapeno-optional
1 bunch kale, chopped
1 c. nopales cactus, chopped
Salt & pepper to taste

Rinse and soak beans overnight. Drain water.
Cook beans as directed on package, adding onions,
garlic, cumin, and chili powder. After about 30
minutes, add in carrots, celery, and tomatoes.
Cook another 30 minutes or so. When beans are
about ready, add in kale and cactus, and cook 5-10
minutes. Season to taste with salt and pepper.
ENJOY!

RAINBOW SALAD

1 box organic mixed greens
½ c. purple cabbage, chopped
½ red skinned apple or fruit of choice, chopped
1 radish, thinly sliced
1 carrot, shredded or chopped
1 stalk celery, chopped
¼ - 1 c. toppings of choice, such as nuts, seeds, or herbs (Anything goes in this salad!)

Mouthgasmic Mango Dressing:
3 honey mangoes or 2 large mangoes in chunks
1 yellow bell pepper in chunks, stems and seeds removed
2 tbsp. raw hemp seeds or raw sesame seeds
1 tbsp. fresh rosemary

Blend dressing ingredients until smooth. Lather onto salad and bask in this Mouthgasmic dining experience! Many thanks to fellow Texan Fully Raw Kristina for this inspired salad!

9

IT'S ALL ABOUT PREVENTION

Protecting yourself from disease is the ticket to good health these days. Socrates said "Let food be thy medicine and medicine be thy food." However, be aware that food also can be our poison. Mother nature has put all of the ingredients we need to stay healthy and heal our bodies in the plant kingdom. Fruits and vegetables have endless phytochemicals and antioxidants, nutrients that protect us from disease. Learn and utilize nature's medicine. It is there for you.

Viruses and other pathogens have become silent killers. From strains of the Epstein-Barr virus to the shingles virus, viruses are wreaking havoc on millions of people's health. Many autoimmune diseases and cancers are viral in nature. Antibiotic-resistant Streptococcus (a bacteria) has become problematic as well. Knowing how to put on your armor and protect yourself is important here! Fruits, vegetables, herbs, and spices are key ingredients towards killing these pathogens. Viruses hate vitamin C! I recommend taking a good quality vitamin C such as Ester C by Pure Encapsulations or Liposomal C by Lipo Naturals. (See chapter 12 for foods high in Vitamin C)

As a nation, we have become seriously deficient in zinc. Protecting yourself by increasing the zinc in your diet is important. Some of the best plant sources of zinc include: (eaten raw is best)

> Cashews
> Coconuts
> Macadamia nuts
> Pecans
> Pine nuts
> Poppy seeds
> Pumpkin seeds
> Sesame seeds
> Spinach
> Sunflower seeds

You can also take a high quality ionic liquid zinc supplement to build your immune system. Good State Ionic Zinc is one of the best on the market. However, all supplements are not created equal; many have toxic fillers. Go to *medicalmedium.com/preferred/supplements* for the best quality supplements on the market. I completely trust this website.

As for heart disease, we live in a country where heart disease has become the norm. As a result, having a cholesterol level of 200 mg/dl is no longer of great concern. In regions where heart disease does not exist, a cholesterol level of 150 mg/dl is considered in the normal range. A low-density lipoprotein (LDL) result between 50 and 70 is ideal. A sure fire way to eliminate and/or reverse heart disease is not to eat foods with cholesterol. Animal products are the *only* foods that contain cholesterol.

As a cardiac nurse, I have seen the pain and suffering my dad and many others have gone through with heart disease. All of the diseases my dad had were man-made, so to speak. To name a few, he had heart disease, hypertension, high cholesterol, type 2 diabetes, and gout, *all* of which are preventable and usually reversible. Know that you have the power to choose differently through your diet and lifestyle choices.

One of my dear friends, who eats only a plant-based diet, recently went to her doctor for a checkup. Her lab work came in and revealed her cardiac risk was a ONE! Her doctor thought there had been a mistake and wanted to recheck her lab. In fact, none of the doctors in the clinic had ever seen this! She had to explain to her doctor that she did not consume *any* cholesterol *or* animal foods in her diet and that was why her numbers were unbelievable!

10

A HEALTHY

BEAUTY TIP

If it is not edible, do not put it on your skin. Our skin is like a sponge that absorbs everything that we put on it. Research has shown that the average woman uses anywhere from 168 to 515 different chemicals DAILY on her body!!! WOW!

Ladies, there are some exceptional organic lines of makeup out there. Please do your research! Coconut oil makes a wonderful skin moisturizer, is edible, and smells great. As for deodorant, we are supposed to perspire! We perspire to release toxins and cool down our bodies. Lathering our armpits with toxic chemicals is not a good idea.

The following is a good recipe for a natural deodorant. This one is my favorite out of all the ones I have tried.

½ c. Natural baking soda
½ c. Organic non-GMO corn starch
4 tbsp. Unrefined coconut oil (melted)
Essential oils:
Lavender - 6 drops
Vetiver - 5 drops
Frankincense/myrrh blend - 5 drops
Rose otto - 7 drops
Tea tree or tulsi - 2 drops
(You can play with different blends of essential oils if some of these are unavailable.)

Mix all ingredients well in a bowl with a fork. Store in a glass jar. Powder those pits and rest assured you will stay fresh all day!

11

GO GREEN

The chemical industry is a HUGE industry in the United States. Toxic chemicals are virtually in almost everything we buy these days. From furniture, carpet, clothing, laundry detergent, dryer sheets, air fresheners, beauty products, to even our water sources, we are inundated with chemicals. It is no wonder why so many people are dying of cancer these days. Our bodies are *very* resilient but we can only tolerate so many toxic products in us!

I encourage you to begin "greening" your home by going through and removing as many toxic chemicals as you can. If you cannot pronounce the ingredients, consider tossing the item, especially if the item has a warning label. There are many websites that can give you tips for a greener home. Some of the products I have replaced in my home for safer options are my cleaning supplies, laundry detergents, soaps, shampoo, deodorant, makeup, plastic containers, feminine products, pesticides, and pet food.

12

WEIGHT LOSS IN THE 21ST CENTURY

Weight loss in the 21st Century is not what it used to be in the 1970's, 80's, and even 90's. Americans have a whole new set of health issues. Obesity is at epidemic proportions in the United States and is increasing each year. Heart disease, cancer, diabetes, and autoimmune diseases are growing exponentially. Children are getting fatty liver disease and what used to be called Type 2 adult onset diabetes. With new fad diets coming out all the time, it has become very confusing to know what to eat anymore and especially how to eat to lose weight.

A few years ago I found myself 15 lbs. over-weight, with a small tire of fat around my waist and elevated liver enzymes. I had a fatty liver and a fatty belly! By reducing the amount of animal products, meats, eggs, oils, and fats in my diet and increasing fruits and vegetables, the weight came right off and the liver enzymes went back to normal.

What most people do not know is that most of the problem lies in our livers. Our livers have a multitude of jobs they perform. The liver holds a VITAL storage of glucose that is available when the body needs it. For instance, when you go for long hours without eating, the liver will release this glucose into the body for energy. This process helps to protect the pancreas and prevents us from getting diabetes.

This glucose storage is like liquid gold. When the storage runs dry, our liver's "filters" get plugged up, leading to unexplained weight gain, diabetes, high blood pressure, and other health issues such as pre-fatty liver and fatty liver disease. Also, when our glucose storage runs out, our adrenal glands are forced to kick in and release adrenaline. This constant adrenal surge is corrosive to our body and wears down the adrenal glands.

The vital glucose reserves in the liver must be replenished. Many studies show that following a low fat, whole food, plant-based diet is the healthiest way to do this. Replenishing glucose reserves can also be achieved by largely reducing the amount of animal proteins, fats, and dairy in the diet. For instance, if you eat animal protein at every meal, try reducing it by eating a small portion of lean protein once a day or every other day (btw, pork is the least healthiest of all meats). Replace these animal proteins and fats with foods such as sweet potatoes, winter squash, and a little avocado, basically lots of fruits, vegetables, beans, lentils, and a few healthy grains like brown rice, millet, and quinoa.

One very important aspect to support the adrenals is to graze often throughout the day, about every two hours or so. Eat well-balanced snacks and meals consisting of foods that contain natural sodium, potassium, and fruit glucose. An example of a balanced snack would consist of apple (fruit glucose), celery stick (natural source of sodium), and dates (natural source of potassium).

One important way to support weight loss is to drink 16 oz. of lemon water every morning upon awakening and throughout the day. This is a safe and gentle way to cleanse the liver. If you are into juicing, a blend of celery, cucumber, and parsley juice is fabulous for liver cleansing. The juice mixture helps to purge the liver of toxins. Other beverages to try are red clover tea (cleans blood and liver), nettle tea, and roasted dandelion tea. These teas are loaded with vital nutrients.

Foods that heal the liver are:
Apples with red skins
Artichokes with hearts
Arugula – has Vitamin C
Asparagus
Berries - high in Vitamin C
Broccoli - Vitamin C (great for liver health)
Butternut Squash
Fresh Dandelion Greens (from your yard, and yes it has Vitamin C also!)
Grapefruit - Vitamin C

Kale –Vitamin C

Oranges - Vitamin C

Spinach –Vitamin C

Other ways to support the liver include jumping on a trampoline or rebounder 10 minutes a day to help with circulation and liver detoxification and using an infrared sauna 15-20 minutes twice a week. Basically moving the body and sweating a little bit.

Along with the liver and adrenals, the thyroid gland is another organ crucial in weight loss. Many people have been diagnosed with thyroid conditions and told they have an autoimmune disease and their bodies are attacking themselves. This is false! Our bodies would never turn on us. In fact, they do everything in their power to protect us and keep us well. Some practitioners and doctors now know most thyroid problems result from the Epstein Barr Virus (EBV) attacking the thyroid, *not* the patients' bodies attacking themselves. When treated with a proper antiviral protocol, the thyroid problem can vanish! For more information, I suggest Anthony William's book *Medical Medium*.

Some healing foods and supplements for thyroid health include:

Ashwaganda
Atlantic dulse (seaweed)
Brazil nuts
Cilantro
Fresh cranberries
Garlic
Hawaiian spirulina
Hemp seeds
Lemon balm tea – antiviral
Licorice root – kills EBV in the thyroid and supports the adrenals
Nascent iodine
Siberian ginseng – for energy
Sprouts
Wild blueberries
Zinc sulfate – antiviral

The key to weight loss in the 21st Century is in supporting these three organs: the liver, the adrenals, and the thyroid. By eating a low-fat, whole food, mostly plant-based diet, this can be done. The bonus in eating this way is that you can eat pretty much all you want, never feel deprived, improve your general health, and watch the weight fall off!

I am grateful we know what we know now. I would have given anything if this information were available for my dad.

13

ACTIVITY, MOVE

THE BODY!

The saying *If you don't use it, you lose it* is true! We must keep these amazing bodies moving and active to sustain our health and mobility. Just like a car, if we let them sit too long, the batteries die, and other things can go wrong. Similarly, our bodies will not perform optimally when we do not care for them properly.

Finding an activity we love is the key. Whether the activity be walking, weightlifting, yoga, or just working on projects around the house, find what suits you and do it...think back to when you were a child and remember what you loved to do. Our bodies typically crave movement so learn to listen to your bodies. They will let you know what they need.

Exercise is very individualized. People in wheelchairs or even bedridden can benefit from exercise. I recently meet a man at the gym who everyone knows as *Papa*. He did not start lifting weights until he was 87 years old, and come to find out he is now 92 years young AND does not look a day over 70.

I asked Papa what was his secret to health and longevity, and this is what he told me.

1. His faith in God
2. Family
3. Positive attitude
4. And a little brandy!

So never think you are "TOO OLD" to do anything! Do whatever you need to get your body moving. Hire a trainer to assist you. Ask a friend to start walking with you or, better yet, take the dog out on a walk.

The times I have felt the best throughout my life was always when I was on a regular exercise program. This was true for my dad as well. He was put on a cardiac rehab exercise program after one of his major heart episodes. He lost weight and was virtually in the best shape of his life! Unfortunately, he quit his exercise and healthy lifestyle program, and…well, you know the rest of the story.

14

RELATIONSHIPS

Our relationships with people, including our significant others, family, friends, and co-workers, are crucial keys to our wellbeing. Many times we may even believe that our happiness depends on other people and how they act. It does not by the way! We are 100% in charge of our own happiness. Finding creative ways to accept and get along with others can be significant. We cannot change them, but we sure can change our minds and perspective on how we view these people in our lives.

There may be that one co-worker who just rubs us wrong. Rather than focusing on their shortcomings, we can change our perspective and begin to look at them in a different light by learning to change our focus from the negative to the positive aspects of that person. For example, if this person were not there in the office with you, your workload could potentially double. How stressed would you feel then?

Finding just one positive aspect to notice about someone and learning to be grateful for that one positive thing can be life changing because what we focus on ALWAYS grows. May we grow each day in gratitude and appreciation for others. It sure beats *hating*!

In our relationships with our significant others, learning to be grateful for that person and focusing on what we love about them can completely change the dynamics of our relationship. Rather than using our precious time and energy focusing on all the "little" things that annoy us, try turning it around and thanking each person for the little things that you appreciate about him or her. Humans just want to be loved and appreciated. Additionally, learning to speak up about our wants and needs from others can be helpful. Believe me, most of us are not mind readers, so clear communication is a must!

Our Number ONE relationship though is truly with ourselves. If we do not love ourselves, how can we possibly love others? Learning to completely love and accept oneself is key! Just a little food for thought…

15

OUR CAREERS

Do what you love and love what you do! We have the choice to choose our career. When I was 18 years old, I felt a deep calling to become a nurse. Throughout my career I have learned how diverse nursing can be. Because I enjoy versatility, I was fortunate to find there are many different paths to take in nursing.

After experiencing many different fields of nursing, being a Wellness Nurse and Nutritional Health Coach is what I now choose to be. If for some reason you dislike the career you chose, then by golly, embark on a new one!

We create our own lives, so getting crystal clear on what we want out of life is important. We can look at our lives as an artist looking at a blank canvas. Just like the artist, we have an infinite number of choices every day.

I like to look at life like a movie, in which I am playing the starring role. Consciously or subconsciously, we are continuously writing the script to our own story. We are all where we are right now because of the choices we have made. If you do not like your "reality show," YOU have the power to change it!

Those unhappy people who blame anyone or anything for their life circumstances are simply not aware of what their true purpose is. If you are in a career that you do not like, there are several options. You can choose to keep doing the same thing and continue to be unhappy, or you can get creative and come up with a way to learn to love your job by changing your perspective. *Or* you can create your dream job. The sky is the limit.

Change takes courage. Begin by writing down and becoming clear on what you want. When you finally realize your life's purpose and love what you do, going to work each day will become a joy.

16

LETTING GO, FORGIVENESS

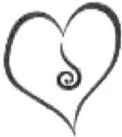

Perhaps you have heard the saying "Let go of the things that no longer serve you." Lack of forgiveness is one of the most toxic emotions we can have. This emotion can cause serious harm to our bodies and minds. Not only does it put us into victim mode and at the mercy of others, it also floods our bodies with toxic emotions and chemicals that harm us. When our bodies get used to staying in fight or flight overdrive, this condition eventually damages our nervous system and causes inflammation in our bodies. Over the years, I have seen this lead to sickness and death.

One tragic story was that of my mother's. She was always vibrant and healthy, until she got breast cancer in her 40's and died at 53 years old. She went to the doctor for a lump in her breast and he told her, "Honey, we are going to have to put the knife to you."

Those very words scared her literally to death. She never saw another doctor, and unfortunately those dreaded words never left her. She took no medications or medical treatments throughout her illness, as she was a practicing Christian Scientist at the time and this religion does not believe in this. My mother also had unresolved emotions that she held onto throughout her life. I think she probably had unrealistic expectations, anger, and resentment toward several family members.

I imagine she also had a difficult time with forgiveness. I truly believe her lack of forgiveness and "letting things go", played a part in her early demise. Harboring anger, fear, and hurts can build up in the body and can sometimes prove to be life threatening.

As has been my experience, I have absolutely no control of what others do and say. But I do certainly have control of how I choose to act or react to them. Learning to "Let it GO" can actually save us. When we forgive, we are not accepting that what happened to us is okay. We are *freeing* ourselves from this toxic burden and releasing the negative hold this has on us. Releasing it, letting it go. Forgive those who have hurt you and move on.

There are many ways to practice forgiveness:

1. Make a list of all the people that you need to forgive, go through the list one person at a time, visualize each person standing in front of you, and say to them "I forgive you." Then burn the list if you so choose.

2. *Ho opono pono* technique. This is a Hawaiian technique that is used by visualizing the person or situation that needs forgiving and saying "I am sorry. Forgive me. Thank you. I love you." Say these words as many times as you need until you feel the burden has lifted. A doctor used this technique with patients in an insane asylum and with miraculous results. He looked at a picture of each person and repeated the saying. Before long

all the people got better and the entire facility was closed down.

3.   Light a candle. Focusing intently on the flame, visualize the person you need to forgive and, when you are ready, say, "I forgive you." I credit my great musician friend Cynthia Jordan for sharing this one.

4.   Lastly, maybe it is YOU who needs forgiving. We can be brutally hard on ourselves at times. Learn to be gentle with yourself and know that you are doing the best that you can. Have compassion for yourself. Have mercy.

Learning to go with the flow of life rather than taking everything personally can be a liberating notion. Because what we resist, persists. The very act of focusing on a problem, adds fuel to it and the problem grows. Well, at least it grows in our minds. Problems are never solved with the same awareness or energy that created them. Shifting our attention to a solution can be all it takes to solve a problem.

17

BE CRYSTAL CLEAR ON WHAT YOU WANT

Focus on what you want, NOT on what you do not want! How many times have we said something to the liking of "Well, I don't want this or I don't want that"? The mere act of focusing on what we DO NOT want can bring that very thing to us!

I actually experienced this first hand. I still laugh today at this story. A number of years ago when I was ready for a new relationship, I decided to write a list of the specific qualities of the man I wanted to be with: dark, wavy hair, hazel eyes, a teacher, someone I can learn from, creative, musically inclined, energetic, fun, and must love Willie Nelson. The list went on, and sure enough a few months later, I met this very man and we soon fell in love. There was only one problem with my list. I made the grave mistake of putting the *ONE* thing on the list that I absolutely did not want in a man, specifically that I DID NOT WANT A PACK RAT. Well, come to find out he not only was a bona fide pack rat, he was even born in the Chinese year of the RAT! He is a total rat, but we love him.

This is how the Universe works: *Ask and you shall receive*! The moral of the story is, be crystal clear on what you want, *NOT* on what you do not want. This notion has been an eye-opening lesson for me to learn. Haters only bring more hate. A war against drugs or terrorism only brings more of that very thing we do not want. Let us choose our battles wisely and learn to say what we truly want in life. Write it down, visualize it, and *imagine* how you will feel when you actually have what you want. Feel that feeling, enjoy that feeling, and watch your dreams come true.

Visualization and "playing pretend" actually works. Give it a try.

18

THE POWER OF THE MIND: FAITH OR FEAR

The power of the mind is truly amazing. Our faith is an integral part of this power we have. Believing in something can either make or break us. I truly believe that our faith in our health and our ability to heal is a crucial part to staying healthy these days. Faith can lead us from darkness to the light. *Believe* and you shall *receive.*

Cases of doctors telling patients they have cancer and have three months to live had been documented. Sure enough, they died in three months, but no cancer was found when the autopsy was done. Many other cases have been noted where patients have been given a terminal diagnosis but they refused to accept that they were going to die, and miraculous healings occurred.

As a nurse I have seen firsthand where people's worst fears come true. Recently, a man I know suddenly became ill with pancreatic cancer, and the doctors told him he only had six weeks to live. He had a history of having diabetes, and come to find out his worst fear was that he would have to get his leg amputated like his mother had. Sure enough, within weeks of his grim diagnosis, his leg started to turn black and he was told that he would have to have it amputated...and this was a man who had previously reversed his diabetes with a healthy diet and lifestyle. His worst *fear* came true.

My father, on the other hand, was in bad health his whole life, but he had a very strong faith and will to live. He did not harbor anger, resentment, or unforgiveness. As I mentioned before, his doctors could not believe he lived as long as he did with his heart condition. He really had a huge heart and will to live.

The early death of both my parents has been my inspiration to search out and learn as much as possible to help others lead a happy and healthy life. Love and a strong faith will set us free from suffering. Anger, fear, resentment, and stress will paralyze us and disease can take over. I believe this. So let us believe with all our hearts that love heals and faith leads our way. Trusting in the process of life, not resisting it, is the key.

Know that the Power of the Mind is an epic life changer.

BELIEVE and you shall *RECEIVE!*

19

THE POWER OF
THE WORD

Our words also have more power than we sometimes realize. Whatever words come after the statement "I AM" becomes our reality. Whether it be "I am doing great!" "I am sick and tired of..." "I hate…" or "I can't stand…" Becoming more conscious of the words that come out of our mouths can made a huge difference in the way we and those around us feel.

Experiments by the late Japanese doctor, Dr. Masaru Emoto, revealed that water responds to the human consciousness and could react to positive thoughts and words spoken to it. When water was spoken to lovingly with the words "I LOVE YOU", the water would form beautiful crystal formations when frozen and examined under a microscope.

Now, when negative words were spoken to the water or death metal music was played to it, the once beautiful water crystals would form into ugly, dark, muddled blobs! The point of the story is that our bodies are made up of about 70% water and respond to how we talk to them and to others. Choose your words wisely.

I believe the obsession with TV and "Hollyweird" (as my friend Reggie DeSoto from Los Angeles used to call it) is actually affecting our health and wellbeing. The fact that we get off on shows about murder and violence just cannot be good for us. Something is just wrong with this picture show! If you choose to watch the tele, try watching comedies or positive programs that uplift you.

Remember, what we focus on grows, and like Papa said, "A positive attitude is one of the most important keys to health, wellness, longevity, and happiness." So not only monitoring our thoughts, but also being mindful of the words we speak can make a world of difference in how we feel.

When I notice my mind wandering into worry mode or negative thoughts, I have several prayers, blessings, and mantras I use to help bring it back into check.

This has been my favorite prayer since I was a little girl. *The LIGHT of God surrounds me, the LOVE of God enfolds me, the POWER of God protects me, and the PRESENCE of God watches over me. Wherever I AM, God IS, and ALL IS WELL.* This little prayer has gotten me through many a situation in my lifetime.

Another favorite is a blessing that is sung at the end of each Kundalini Yoga class. *May the longtime sun shine upon you. All Love surround you, and the pure Light within you, guide your way on.*

Finally, I learned some great mantras when I studied yoga. *Sat Nam* means *Truth is my identity*. May we always live and speak our truth. *Wahe Guru* means *Wonderful Teacher,* in which teacher refers to God. To me it means God is Great!

One of my favorite Bible quotes comes from Matthew 19:26, which states, *"With God all things are possible."*

I prefer to add, *"I AM with God, and ALL things are possible."* I will say this aloud or to myself as many times as needed to calm my mind and restore my faith.

20

THE POWER OF GRATITUDE

Another great practice to help get in a better frame of mind is practicing gratitude. Having an *Attitude of Gratitude* rocks. I first started using a gratitude meditation when I began teaching yoga classes. During the relaxation part of our yoga practice, we always take a few minutes to come to our hearts and give thanks for all that we have, including one another, our families, our friends, and our community.

An additional integral part of a gratitude practice is to allow ourselves to feel the actual feeling of gratitude. In feeling the feeling of gratitude for all that we have, we promote positive, healing chemicals to be released into our body. These healing chemicals allow us to *feel good* and help our bodies maintain homeostasis.

One more great way to practice gratitude is starting and ending the day with gratitude. This can be done by keeping a journal and writing down all the things which you are grateful for *and* the reasons why you are grateful for them. Or just taking time to think about or verbalize all that you are grateful for.

Prayer also is an excellent way to give thanks for all that we have. Blessing and giving thanks for our food before eating is a wonderful practice. Always remember that what we focus on grows, so how about growing each and every day in gratitude for all that we have. Thank you all for taking the time to read this today. *I AM* Grateful!

21

THE HEALING POWER
OF MUSIC

Music has been known as the universal language. Personally, I cannot imagine a day in my life without music! In more recent years, I have become more conscious of the music I listen to and how it makes me feel. When I was younger, I would listen to music that would evoke strong emotions in me, whether they were positive or negative, I did not pay much attention. Now, I choose music that is more positive, lifts my spirits, and makes me feel good. Remember what happened to the water when the death metal music was played? I will pass on that – no thanks!

I was recently in Mexico visiting my family and met an amazing young man named Mauro. Mauro is a renowned concert pianist, and he told me a great story about how music is like medicine. An older gentleman and dear friend of his had recently been diagnosed with a terminal illness and was dying. Towards the end of his life, the man's pain levels had become unbearable. All he could think about was how bad the pain was. Then an idea came to him to have his caregiver put on his favorite piece of music, a classic called *Hansel and Gretel*. As soon as the music began, his focus shifted to the music and his pain began to subside. Before long he was no longer focused on the pain and it went away. Music helped him relax and days later he died peacefully. The family requested Mauro play this same piece of music at his funeral and he graciously accepted.

Mauro told another story about music and mind over matter. A while back he had fallen and severely broke his hand. He went to the best hand doctor in the area and was told that, due to the location and severity of the break, he would no longer be able to play the piano. Mauro said he never believed those words for a moment. He was 100% confident that he would heal and continue to play. All he had ever known was music and this is how he made a living. He knew within his heart he had no other choice but to focus on healing and continue playing piano. Mauro showed me his hand and there was a definite deformity. He then sat down at the piano and began to play one of the most beautiful pieces I have ever heard.

Another amazing inspirational musician is my dear friend Cynthia Jordan. Her mission statement is *"To Heal the World with Music."* She has composed numerous songs, albums, and musicals over the years. She never ceases to amaze me how the music keeps flowing out of her. From her #1 country hit "Jose Cuervo," to her Christmas music, to her Celtic tunes, her music has truly healed many on this planet.

Consider turning off the TV and turning on your favorite music. Better yet, take up playing an instrument, singing, or dancing.

22

JUST BREATHE...DECOMPRESS!

Stress has become rampant in our society. Since the beginning of the Industrial Revolution, the amount of information being thrown at us each day is unbelievable! If you watch the news, you cannot help but notice all the text information flying across the bottom of the screen on top of all the dreadful stories.

Life can be flat out stressful, and we now know stress is a MAJOR risk factor to disease...or "Dis – Ease" as I like to call it.

Conscious breathing is a simple technique that can be used any time of the day to relax and decompress from all the craziness around us. Just taking in one deep breath can even prevent a blowout with our loved ones. Stopping for a moment and taking a deep breath helps us regroup our emotions and ACT, rather than REACT, to someone or something.

Dr. Andrew Weil teaches the 4 – 7 – 8 breathing technique that benefits the body and mind in many ways. This breathing helps to calm the sympathetic nervous system, bringing us out of "fight or flight" mode, and into the parasympathetic nervous system, the "rest and digest" mode. Simply relax the body by breathing in a long, deep breath through the nose to the count of 4, then hold the breath in for the count of 7, and finally exhale slowly through the mouth for 8 counts. Doing about 5 cycles of this breathing several times a day can do wonders for us, including bringing our bodies into homeostasis, letting go of stress, and even promoting weight loss.

If you look at a baby breathe, they are breathing correctly. When a baby inhales, their belly expands, and when they exhale the belly decompresses. Somehow in our busy lives, we have forgotten how to breathe. Place your hand on your belly. As you slowly inhale, allow your belly to expand outwards, and as you exhale, gently press on the belly as the air leaves your lungs. This is our diaphragm at work; the diaphragm is one of the largest muscles in the body. We tend to inhale and stick our chest out and suck our bellies in as our shoulders come up towards our ears. This is backwards. Just relax your shoulders and chest and let your diaphragm do the work. It may take a little practice to get the hang of it, but the benefits are well worth it.

The nice thing about conscious breathing is you can literally do it anywhere. I like to practice when I am driving or in heavy traffic. Instead of reacting to being stuck in traffic, I relax and just practice my deep breathing techniques. Breathe in, breathe out.

There are many ways to reduce stress. Some of my favorites include getting out in nature, exercising, playing with my animals, listening to music, and spending quality time with friends. One of my all-time favorite ways to relieve stress and tension is taking hot baths with essential oils and sea salts. Lavender is a *lovely* essential oil for promoting relaxation and decreasing stress. Hot baths are not only extremely relaxing, but when we are in this relaxed state, brilliant ideas and revelations can come to us! In the same way as with meditation, when our minds are relaxed, ideas and answers often come to us. These methods are wonderful ways to get grounded. Find what relaxes you, and do it often. Schedule this YOU time into your calendar if needed.

23

GET SOME REST!

Lastly, get some rest! This is something we tend to overlook and shortchange ourselves. When we take the time to sleep eight or more hours a night, our bodies have adequate time to rest and restore at a deeper level. This is the time when our bodies are working at a cellular level to detox, restore, and heal themselves. Our minds are at work too; as we go into dreamtime, our subconscious mind sorts out all our "stuff."

Our dreams can even have messages for us. One friend says that oftentimes he will wake up in the morning with a solution to an issue he was having. Keeping a dream journal and writing down your dreams as soon as you wake up can be a helpful practice.

At a recent Wellness and Nutrition class I was teaching to a group of young teenage girls, one girl told me she had to drink coffee in the morning just to get up and get going. Come to find out her schedule was so packed that it was sometimes midnight before she finished her homework and could get to sleep. What does this tell us about how stressful our lives have become nowadays, even for children.

Many people's minds are so wired at night that they have a hard time falling asleep. I recommend finding ways to relax in the evening and unwind. Once again a hot bath with sea salts, essential oils, and candles is a great way to relax the body and mind. A massage is also a wonderful way to relax. The human touch is so important for us, make sure to get in your hugs and kisses whenever possible! Listening to relaxing music or meditating can also be helpful ways to unwind in the evenings. Reading a good book always helps me to relax, unwind, and fall asleep.

Whenever possible hold off on screen time from computers, phones, and TV at least an hour before going to sleep. Recent studies have found that the bright lights emitted from these devices interrupt the production of melatonin, the hormone that helps regulate sleep and wake cycles. Dimming the lights in the house when the sun goes down can be helpful as well. Removing all electronics from the bedroom will help facilitate a good night's rest. This includes Wi-Fi, computers, and any devices that emit light. Have the room as dark as possible. The bedroom should be used as a place for sleep and intimacy only.

Keeping the bedroom clean, de-cluttered, and decorated nicely will help encourage a peaceful night's rest as well. Plants in the home and bedroom will help purify the air quality in your home. Your body and mind will surely thank you for taking steps to ensure a good night's sleep.

24

SUMMARY

Looking back, the times when I was the happiest and healthiest was when I was incorporating these healthy tips into my life. Commit to discovering the healthiest you possible! Surround yourself with friends and family who support your happiness and well-being. Work to build strong relationships, focusing on quality family and friend time. We tend to be happier and healthier when our relationships with others are in order.

Find a health care practitioner who listens to you. If you currently are not satisfied with your doctor or practitioner, consider finding a new one. You may want to look for an integrative or functional medicine doctor, one who is trained in getting to the root cause of your issues. Treating symptoms with drugs does not correct the existing problem.

Eat *real food* y'all! Add in more fresh fruits and vegetables and drink more water. Move your body by staying active. Exercise your body and mind. Be open-minded and try out new things. Studies on healthy centenarians (those over 100 years old) from around the world found this group to be future oriented. They were always making plans and looking forward to each new day. The centenarians enjoyed active lives; many loved nature and gardening and were surrounded by a supportive community.

Choose a career you are passionate about and love or decide to learn to love your current work. Learn to forgive yourself and others. Let go of any grudges and go with the flow of life.

Focus on what you want, NOT on what you do not want out of life. Have faith and know that positive thoughts and a positive attitude will create positive outcomes. An Attitude of Gratitude will attract more good things for which you will be grateful.

Enjoy music, song, and the dance of life. Get out in nature as often as possible and catch a sunrise or sunset. Gaze at the stars under the moonlight. Get your hands and feet in the dirt and do some gardening. Tend to Mother Earth and she will always share her gifts with you.

Lastly, just breathe, relax, and get your Zzzzz's! Consider hiring a health coach. Prevention and health coaching is going to be the wave of the future. It has to be. From the bottom of my heart, I wish you Health and Happiness always!

25

SOME OF MY FAVORITES

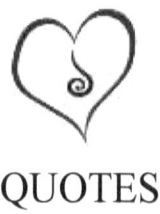

QUOTES

What we focus on grows

What we resist, persists

Focus on what you want, NOT on what you do not want

Yesterday is dead and gone, and tomorrow's out of sight. ~Kris Kristofferson

Be here now

We are spiritual beings having a human experience.

Believe and you shall receive

I AM with God and ALL things are possible

Happiness is a choice

Let it go

It is what it is

Have an attitude of gratitude

Just breathe

If you want more, give more

"Love like your life depends on it, cuz it does."
~Michael Franti

"Never finish a negative statement; reverse it
immediately and wonders will happen
in your life." ~Dr. Joseph Murphy
(My brother was named after this man)

"Whether you think you can, or think you can't, you are right." ~Henry Ford

If you keep doing the same ole things, you'll keep getting the same ole results

AUTHORS & BOOKS

Louise Hay - *You Can Heal Your Life*

Anthony Williams - *Medical Medium* and *Life-Changing Foods*

Christiane Northrup, M.D. – *Goddesses Never Age*

Guru Singh - *Buried Treasures*

Paramahansa Yogananda - *Autobiography of a Yogi*

Esther and Jerry Hicks - *Ask and It Is Given*

Dr. Joseph Murphy - *The Power of Your Subconscious Mind*

Emmett Fox - *The Golden Key*

T. Collin Campbell, PhD - *The China Study*

Leanne Campbell, PhD - *The China Study All-Star Collection Cookbook*

Lindsay S. Nixon – *The Happy Herbivore - Guide to Plant Based Living & Cookbook*

Kristina Carrillo-Bucaram - *The Fully Raw Diet*

Patch Adams, *M.D. – House Calls*

Willie Nelson and Turk Pipkin - *The Tao of Willie* (I can't leave out my favorite Texan)

INSPIRATIONAL MUSICIANS

Michael Franti

Pele Juju

Ziggy Marley

Jason Mraz

Willie Nelson and son Lukas Nelson

Cynthia Jordan

Deva Premal

Snatam Kaur

Guru Singh

Santana

Stevie Wonder

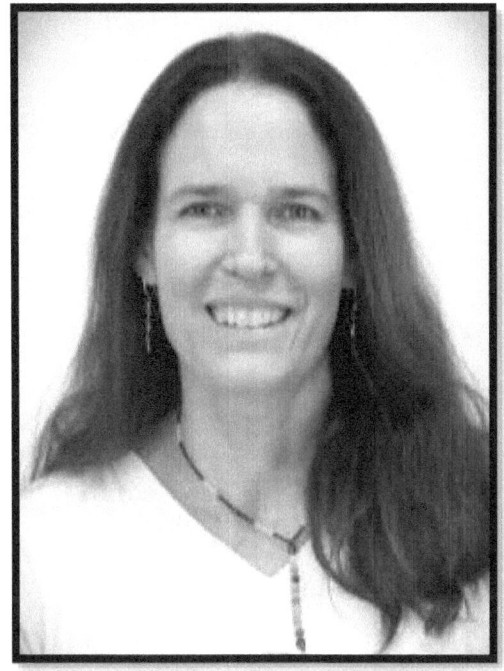

Photo by M.W. "Mike" Erb

Alicia Lown, R.N. has been working in the health care industry for over 25 years. As a Certified Integrative Nutrition and Health Coach, her passion lies in helping others to live happy, healthy lives. This interest began after seeing both her parents' lives cut short due to heart disease and cancer. She then made it her life's mission to dedicate herself to discovering the keys to Health & Happiness in the 21st century.